OIL PULLING

Cleansing Therapy to Reverse Gum Disease & Heal the Body

Sonja Y. Larsen

Oil Pulling

Copyright © 2015 by Sonja Larsen

All rights reserved. No part of this book may be reproduced or transmitted in any form or by any means without written permission from the author.

ISBN 978-1512039979

Printed in USA

Disclaimer

It is an absolute condition of the sale of this book that you consult with your doctor or health care practitioner before practicing any of the methods described in this book. This book is for educational purposes only and is not intended to treat, cure or prevent any condition or disease. The author shall not be held responsible or liable for any loss or damage from any suggestion or information contained in this book.

Other Books by Sonja Y. Larsen:

Oil Belly, Flat Belly: Burn Belly Fat with Oils and Fats from Your Kitchen

Superdrinks for Superhumans: 50 Healthy Recipes to Fuel Productivity and Workouts

Why You Need To Read This Book

Oil pulling will allow you to perform a daily cleansing ritual that you will come to love once you get the hang of it. You can experience a glorious transformational shift in the way you look and feel. It's simply about becoming beautiful from the inside out. When you're cleansed and all bodily systems are working properly, it shows on the outside.

Oil pulling can be a bit messy at first. And the health benefit does not happen overnight. But once you repeat this ritual for 21 days, you'll never want to go without.

I once went without. I got a wild hair and decided I was "pretty healthy" and stopped oil pulling for two weeks. Wow. What a disaster. First, my nose and throat developed a ton of mucous. I was constantly trying to swallow it and keep it on lockdown so no one would see how excessively snotty I was. I suppose it was a cold or a flu–something I hadn't experienced in years.

Then I started gaining all this weight. It was maddening, because I go to the gym and workout all the time. How could I be gaining weight at record pace?

My skin looked dull and had lost some of its luster. A few more months of non-oil-pulling laziness, and I would graduate from funeral director to gravedigger.

The worst part was that some tooth pain kicked in. I had never had a single cavity before. But I did have a very ~~sexy~~ handsome dentist tell me many years ago that a single tooth of mine was on the brink of decay, and to take care of that tooth very well. And so I took care of my little snaggletooth, and was able to ward off any cavities for years.

However, when I stopped oil pulling, my tooth sensitivity worsened, and I worried–no, panicked–that I might have to go to the dentist for my tooth. I didn't have any dental insurance, and had no desire to experience severe pain, coupled with severe loss of money.

What the heck happened? It was because I had stopped oil pulling. I knew oil pulling worked, but I figured I could stop and that I was "good to go," after having pulled for many years. Boy, was I wrong.

I needed to keep up the practice if I was to have good health. I am happy to report that all is back to normal–lost the extra pounds, coughed up all the mucous in a matter of days, and made it through that cavity scare. I'm back in the game.

Oil pulling is an ancient Ayurvedic method of cleansing. It benefits the body by pulling toxins from your mouth. Secondly, the oil is absorbed by the tongue, under the tongue, the inside of the cheeks, and the gums. This process is used by the body to heal infected areas. During this exchange, the healing properties of the oils saturate the areas closest to the mouth, like the throat and chest. And then they work their way down to the rest of the body. Essentially, oil pulling is a way to anoint the entire body with oil from the inside. The most immediate area that the oil heals is the mouth itself.

After oil pulling, people have claimed to experience improvements in:

- o Weight Loss
- o Candida Overgrowth
- o Acne
- o Teeth Whitening
- o Asthma
- o Eczema
- o Colitis
- o Chron's Disease

- Irritable Bowel Syndrome (IBS)
- Periodontal Disease
- Bleeding Gums
- Cavities
- Gingivitis
- Hemorrhoids
- Chronic Fatigue

Are you suffering from any of these health issues? If so, then you better give oil pulling a try.

You have made a good decision to read this book. You will be so excited about getting started on this simple, inexpensive home therapy, that you will be knocking people over to get to the oil shelf at the supermarket.

Note: If you are in Desperation Mode and your teeth are getting ready to fall out, skip down to Chapter 3, QUICK!

Table of Contents

Introduction 11

Chapter One:
What the Heck is Oil Pulling 13

Chapter Two:
The Many Benefits of Oil Pulling 19

Chapter Three:
The Teeth and Gums
Desperation Mode 23

Chapter Four:
Step-by-Step How to Do it
Best Oils to Use 29

Chapter Five:
What About Side Effects
Emotions During Detox 41

Sources 46

Bonus Jumpstart Cleanse 49

Last Thoughts 53

One Last Thing 55

About the Author &
Excerpt from Next Book 57

Introduction

The reason I began my oil pulling journey was because I was experiencing inflammation in the intestines and had frequent problems digesting food. I'm a serious foodie, and it seemed like all my favorite foods were being taken away from me. The list of things I could not eat was growing and growing. It was ridiculous. Soon I'd be down to water and celery sticks. I also had problems taking a long deep breath, and had mysteriously developed pulsatile tinnitus in my right ear.

I thought I was already healthy because I went to the gym 6-7 days a week. But exercise isn't everything. It doesn't get rid of happy hour. Some people believe that if they sweat it out at the gym the following day, then it's all good. Margaritas and chicken wings all night, wheezing and hi-fives in the morning. This is a fallacy. And it's a fantasy.

I made several changes to my lifestyle. I stopped nearly all alcohol intake, and started shopping for whole, unprocessed foods. Then I acquired several habits–oil pulling, juicing, consuming teas instead of coffee, using healthy oils, among a few other things.

Once I began a steady morning routine of oil pulling, I noticed small changes. My digestion improved, I could take deeper breaths, my skin was developing a glow, and an unexpected benefit: I started losing weight. I was reborn. And you will be too.

I know this sounds crazy, but I feel and look younger every year. I have way more energy than I did in my twenties and thirties, and I love to share how old I am with complete strangers–just to see their reaction. I love to take care of myself, and I have a few tricks up my sleeve. Oil pulling is one of my best-kept secrets. I have been oil pulling since 2008, and have achieved fantastic results. I'm finally ready to share my secret.

Chapter One

What the Heck is Oil Pulling?

Oil pulling is a technique used to simultaneously pull toxins from the body and replace them with the healing benefits of healthful oils. The practice has been known to alleviate:

- Migraines
- Headaches
- Arthritis
- Inflammation
- Respiratory Problems
- Crohn's Disease and Colitis
- Sinus Congestion
- Allergies

These are just a few diseases which have been documented in a 1996 survey published in a Southern Indian newspaper, Andhra Jyoti. Don't worry about pronouncing the name of the newspaper. Just know that out of 1041 people surveyed, 89% (927 people) reported that oil pulling cured one or more of their diseases. Only a mere 11% (114) reported no benefit.

The survey included the following:

- Pains in the body – 758 cases
- Respiratory system – 191 cases
- Skin – 171 cases
- Digestive system – 155 cases
- Elimination – 137 cases
- Joints – 91 cases

- Heart and Circulation – 74 cases
- Blood Sugar – 56 cases
- Hormones – 21 cases
- Miscellaneous – 72 cases

This newspaper survey is perhaps the most well-known oil pulling publication today, documenting the stories of hundreds of people and their experiences with oil pulling. It contains actual names, dates and conditions of people who had life-threatening diseases and less-serious conditions. Less serious conditions include:

- Weight Loss
- Clear Skin from Acne
- Wrinkle Treatment
- Help with Dry Skin

Oil pulling has its roots in Ayurvedic medicine. It is a cleansing practice that dates back thousands of years. It had been practiced regularly by Indians, but a Ukrainian doctor named Dr. Karach brought it to the Western world in 1992, by sharing it with his fellow doctors in a presentation to the Ukranische-Union of the Oncologists and Bacteriologists. He claimed that his own blood cancer had been completely cured by using the simple oil pulling technique daily. Don't you wish you had a doctor like that—one that looked at natural remedies and didn't automatically throw a bottle of pills at your head?

The Basics of Oil Pulling

Oil pulling is achieved by swishing oil in the mouth for 15-20 minutes and spitting it out into the toilet or trash bin. Does 15-

20 minutes sound like a long time? Don't fret. Once you get the hang of it, you'll want to pull for an hour straight. Family members will be begging you to spit the oil out just so they can talk to you. Just walk around the house and do all the things you would normally do, and time will fly by.

A toilet is used with sesame oil and a trash bin is used with coconut oil, because of the amount of living microscopic bacteria contained in the spit-oil mixture. If you were to use the sink to discard your oil, you would need to bleach it afterward and that would be too much work for your pretty dazzle-hands.

Sesame oil will flush fine, but coconut oil will solidify and clog pipes, so use the trash for spitting. Follow these easy steps to achieve success with oil pulling:

1. Pour cold-pressed oil into a tablespoon. Using a Chinese soup spoon is the easiest way to avoid spillage, but you do not need to fill the tablespoon completely. If you are just beginning oil pulling, you will want to have a smaller, more controllable amount of oil in your mouth. You may want to increase the amount as you get used to oil pulling and if you have a larger mouth. If you have a smaller mouth or you are just beginning oil pulling, stick with about 1/2 to 3/4 tablespoon of oil.

2. Spoon the oil into your mouth.

3. Swish oil in your mouth. Be sure to hit any problem areas, like sensitive teeth, or a bleeding gum area. Do not swallow the oil.

4. Spit out oil into trash or toilet. Oil will have turned into a white foamy liquid by now. Really take your time spitting into the toilet–try to find a private toilet where you can gag and cough up mucous as you spit the oil out. If you use coconut oil, spit it out into a trash bin, as many have reported that the oil can solidify and clog pipes.

5. Rinse and gargle your mouth with a handful of water. This step is to rinse away some of the bacteria and parasites before sticking your toothbrush in your mouth.

6. Brush your teeth and tongue well. Take your time brushing both your teeth and tongue. Remember, a numerous amount of parasites have been there, so you want to saturate the mouth and destroy them. Get 'em all.

7. Drink one or two 8-oz glasses of water. This serves multiple purposes which we will discuss later.

8. Enjoy the benefits of oil pulling!

These are the basic steps of oil pulling. For more in-depth instructions, feast on Chapter Four.

This book was created to help you maintain a successful oil pulling venture. If you follow the guidance in this book, and you continue oil pulling daily for a minimum of 2-3 months, you may begin to see small changes in your body. Everyone is different, so we all respond differently to treatments. But oil pulling is one of the most cost-effective additions to your daily routine that could ultimately change your life.

If you suffer from a serious condition, you have little to lose with this detoxification method, since there are little to none known side effects. Even if you are not afflicted with any certain disease, oil pulling can be an important means for prevention, and give you a highly-desirable glow. Because the method continuously removes bacteria from your body on the daily basis, your chances of avoiding illness are greater than if you practiced no daily output of bacteria. Simply put, it is a daily detox method.

A common mistake of newcomers to the oil pulling practice, is that they do not give oil pulling much of a chance. In order to see the slightest results of oil pulling, you must oil pull daily for a minimum of 2-3 months. Be prepared to go through your first bottle of oil (depending on size) and to need to buy more to get through the first couple months.

If you discredit oil pulling because it is simply too messy or doesn't work in 1-2 weeks, you are short-changing yourself on benefits that could improve both the quality and length of your life. There is no fast road to good health.

Oil pulling is an ongoing process which is part of a healthy lifestyle. Browse the knowledge-base provided in this book as often as you like during your beginning stages of oil pulling, for support and reassurance on this great addition to your health and wellness routine.

Chapter Two

The Many Benefits of Oil Pulling

Oil pulling benefits the body by exchanging fluids. The oil assists in pulling toxins from your mouth, firstly. Secondly, a small amount of oil is absorbed by the tongue, under the tongue, the inside of the cheeks, and the gums. This is used by the body to heal infected areas. During this exchange, the healing properties of specific oils begin to work the areas closest to the mouth. Essentially, oil pulling is a way to anoint the body from the inside. The most immediate area that the oil heals is the mouth itself.

Swishing Action Creates Bile

One of the most interesting things about oil pulling is that the masticating movement of the mouth gives the liver the perception that it is time to digest food. The liver then produces bile, which helps decrease toxicity. It is like tricking the liver into processing a meal, but there is no food, because you're swishing on an empty stomach. So it is going to process items you already ate, but didn't digest and eliminate very well. Yep, even the stuff you really didn't want to eat: hard-to-read food ingredients, dust, bacteria, pet hair...you name it. Liver trickery!

Dental Benefits of Oil Pulling

The oil can be used to pull bad bacteria away from decaying teeth and gums, and can also be used in a preventative manner.

The act of building up saliva in the mouth helps to break down bacteria. Oil pulling specifically targets bad bacteria in the mouth, assisting with:

- Decaying teeth
- Tooth Sensitivity
- Gingivitis
- Periodontal Disease
- Bleeding Gums

Be sure to clear between teeth with a strand of dental floss before beginning oil pulling if there's an area you specifically want to work on. Flossing the areas beforehand will ensure the oil's passage between your teeth. The oil will penetrate all around the teeth, into the gums, and tongue. Depending on the number of bacteria in your mouth and the amount of work the oil needs to complete, the oil will eventually make its way to the throat area. If there is a lot of bacteria and mucous in your mouth, your oil pulling efforts will go to your mouth only, as it will not be able to travel very far. This is totally fine. The oil pulling is working, and it needs to start somewhere. It may take a span of several months to reach beyond the mouth, but it will happen if you pull religiously and do not skip days.

See Chapter Three for an in-depth look at the teeth and gums.

Allergies, Sinusitis, and Breathing

One of the most immediate benefits of daily oil pulling is the ability to clear much of the mucous away from the nose and throat, making it easier to breathe. A good oil pulling session which clears air passage ways will give you a fresh, energized feeling with which to start your day. As mentioned previously, the oil begins pulling parasites and bacteria from the mouth, works its way to the throat and chest after several months. As the oil works its way down through your body, it targets bacteria, pulling it and drawing it up into your mouth, accompanied by a plethora of phlegm.

Skin

As the oil works its way from your mouth to the rest of your head, it begins to assist in the overall circulation of blood. Increased circulation in the facial area will mean that you may notice a difference in:

- Skin Tone
- Acne
- Wrinkles
- Texture or Softness
- Glow
- Eczema
- Rosacea
- Psoriasis

Because the face encompasses the mouth, you will notice effects on the face within a few weeks. First, your skin will detox. If your skin has a lot of underlying bacteria, or this is the first time you are detoxing, you will notice that your skin breaks out into a rash or zits, right off the bat. Don't worry, and don't stop! This simply means that you are detoxing, and it will go away. Your skin cells completely renew themselves after 30 days, so you will not be "stuck" with this condition. Rather, you will find that your skin will eventually be softer, and adopt a brighter, glowing tone.

Oil pulling may also help delete fine lines and prevent wrinkles because of the moisture provided through the oil, from within. Numerous people have also reported improvement in more serious skin conditions and irritations like Eczema, Rosacea, and Psoriasis.

Weight Loss with Oil Pulling

The oil eventually reaches the lungs, kidneys, liver, and colon, working to clear mucous and toxins. The result is that your organs can function better because they are not impaired by parasites, bacteria, and a cloud of phlegm. When your liver is clear to remove toxins, and your intestines contain minimal parasites and candida, your organs will be able to do their job of eliminating food waste. This is when desired weight loss occurs. Not too shabby of a side effect, is it?

Weight loss is a well-known benefit of oil pulling. However, the weight loss tends to be very gradual and is not a speedy way to lose weight. So, do not look to oil pulling to lose quick massive poundage. Rather, consider the inevitable weight loss as a bonus to your overall health.

Chapter Three

The Teeth and Gums

There are a great many advantages to oil pulling for oral health. Some people argue that oil pulling is a hoax, because you can just brush and floss. However, oil pulling should not be used instead of professional dental cleanings, screenings, teeth brushing, and flossing. Rather, it should be used *in conjunction with* traditional and professional dental care. For instance, before oil pulling, you should floss to ensure that the oil has a clear passageway between the teeth. And after oil pulling, it is extremely important that you brush.

Greater care needs to be taken when it comes to dental care. Have you wondered why you still get cavities, fillings, and root canals, even though you brush, floss, and go to your routinely scheduled dental visits? Practicing routine traditional care is simply not enough. It is for the same reason why you still get sick, even though you did your routine annual exams and made regular visits to see your doctor.

You need to take more action to prevent disease and decay. Showing up for a professional dentist cleaning and brushing does not prevent major and minor dental work for most people. Look to oil pulling as a supplemental preventative measure.

Pulled toxins include, but are not limited to:

- o Mercury and other chemicals
- o Candida (thrush)
- o Bacteria

Gingivitis & Periodontal/Gum Disease

Because the oil targets the gum, under the gum, and between the gum and tooth, oil pulling has been reported to help those afflicted with Gingivitis and Periodontal Disease. See "Sources" near the end of this book for specific dental research studies and personal testimonials.

As receding gums collect bacteria and debris, the disease advances into eventual tooth loss. Oil pulling has been used to maintain healthy gums, and clear away bacteria, so it's no wonder why many have claimed improvement to their oral health.

Gingivitis is a condition where bacteria accumulates between the tooth and the gum. The bacteria causes the teeth to become red and inflamed, as it begins to break down healthy tissue and even bone. The bacteria can be very difficult to clear away, as it is tucked away in a little "pocket."

The pocket acts as a barrier between the tooth and the gum and will play a key role in pulling the gum away from the tooth. This is what is commonly referred to as "receding gums." Gums will recede and if left untreated, the disease will advance to periodontal disease.

Gum Disease Symptoms:

- Gums bleed after brushing
- Bad breath
- Red or inflamed gums
- Loose teeth
- Receding gums, or pockets between tooth and gum

People have reported significant change when using oil pulling to combat gum disease. The first thing people tend to mention is that their gums feel "tighter." Oil pulling has even been known to reverse Gingivitis. Sometimes people notice that their teeth are not as loose, and that their gums look healthier and shinier.

In a published researched study conducted by Asokan S, Emmadi P, and Chamundeswari R. to examine whether plaque-induced gingivitis could be reduced by oil pulling, researchers found oil pulling helpful in reversing Gingivitis. They said that the patients "showed a reduction in the plaque index, modified gingival scores, and total colony count of aerobic microorganisms in the plaque of adolescents with plaque-induced gingivitis."

What does that mean in *Engrish*? It means someone's dental situation got a whole lot better from oil pulling.

Desperation Mode

1. Begin a morning routine of oil pulling. See Chapter Four, "Step-by-step, How to Do It," for useful instructions.

2. Continue dentist visits. You'll need to be sure that your oil pulling is working and it helps if a professional can confirm. It's very important not to let your Gingivitis advance to periodontal disease.

3. Add 2-4 drops of Oil of Oregano. This is a way to "supercharge" your oil pulling routine. Be sure to encase the oil of oregano into the coconut or sesame oil first before putting it in your mouth. Oil of Oregano is a very powerful oil, and you won't want it touching every surface of your mouth without the coconut or sesame oil. That will make you go cray-cray. It is not to be used daily, but only in times of desperation!

4. Add one 30-50 mg gel capsule of CoQ10 to the mix. Dr. Bruce Fife, author of Oil Pulling Therapy (another excellent oil pulling reference) recommends emptying the gel capsule directly into the mouth and then spooning your coconut/sesame oil plus oil of oregano mixture into your mouth.

5. Continue flossing and brushing. Don't skimp on the other stuff. Oil pulling is an add-in to the rest of your oral care.

6. Use Clove Oil throughout the day directly on tooth/gum pain. Clove oil alleviates tooth pain. Cloves themselves are good at destroying parasites, so it's good to add clove spice to your food or drinks daily too. Just remember that clove oil shouldn't be used instead of the dentist. Don't end up masking your pain indicator so much that you don't notice deterioration of your teeth and gums. If the teeth are getting worse and worse, get thee to thy dentist.

Overgrowth of Candida (Thrush)

Thrush (oropharyngeal candidiasis) occurs when an overgrowth of Candida albicans builds in the mouth. Candida overgrowth is simply when too much yeast is in the mouth and body. The classic symptom is a white-coated tongue. Oil pulling will help fight yeast as both sesame oil and coconut oils are antifungal. If you have thrush, you will most likely benefit from oil pulling. There is no danger with using the oil pulling method to remove candida.

It is much safer than using Gentian Violet to cure thrush, which is a known carcinogen. We should just rename it "Gently Violent." You want thrush gone, but you do not want to end up with oral cancer. It kind of defeats its own purpose, doesn't it? So try oil pulling and stay away from the Gentian Violet "cure".

Here's what to do for Thrush/Candida:

1. Begin a morning routine of oil pulling. Hit up Chapter Four for the step-by-step guide.

2. Consider adding 1-2 drops of oil of oregano to your oil, on occasion. Oil of oregano is a strong anti-fungal. Add a drop to your main oil (sesame or coconut) before placing in the mouth. It is not to be used regularly, but only in times of desperation!

3. Do not use commercial toothpaste. Your chemicalized toothpaste is most likely contributing to your thrush. Instead, use 100% baking soda, or a 50-50% combination of baking soda and sea salt.

With a steady routine of oil pulling, you will experience a cleaner mouth, and will conquer your infections. Keep pulling, and be patient.

Chapter Four

Step-By-Step: How to Do it (And do it Well)

Are you curious about how to do oil pulling and anxious to get started?

Here's what to do:

1. Floss any areas of the mouth that you especially want to work on. Oil pulling works by saturating the gums and teeth, so be sure to clear the areas of plaque and broccoli to make it easy for the gums to absorb. Once you have completed your flossing, follow step 2, below.

2. Pour oil into a tablespoon. Using a whole tablespoon is easiest to avoid spillage, however you do not need to fill the tablespoon completely. If you are just beginning oil pulling, you will want a smaller, controllable amount of oil in your mouth. You may want to increase the amount as you become accustomed to oil pulling and/or you have a larger-sized mouth. If you have a smaller mouth or you are just beginning oil pulling, stick with about 1/2 to 3/4 tablespoon oil. A set of Chinese soup spoons will work very well here, because they usually measure 1 tablespoon. Use these to ladle the oil into your mouth easily without spilling. These can be purchased inexpensively in sets so that you will always have a clean one available.

If you are using coconut oil, you will need to get a small chunk with a regular metal tablespoon and just place it in your mouth. It will melt after about 30 seconds, and then you can resume oil pulling as normal.

3. Spoon the oil into your mouth. Give it a little slurp at the end to get the last bit.

4. Swish oil in your mouth. Be sure to work on any "problem areas", like sensitive teeth, or a bleeding gum area. One of the best times to oil pull is when you feel like you might be coming down with something. If you already have a cold or allergies and feel the need to sneeze, place a finger under your nose. If you still need to sneeze, move quickly to the kitchen sink. This tends to be the best place to sneeze. Unfortunately, you will lose your oil. But at least you will be able to clean up the mess easier than if you had sneezed down, on, and all around your toilet and bathroom walls. Another great way to keep from messing up anything is to carry a big rag/towel around the house with you, just in case. Make sure you disinfect everything very well after a sneeze occurs.

5. Spit out oil into toilet (or trash bin if you are using coconut oil). Oil will have turned into a white foamy saliva liquid by now. Really take your time spitting into the toilet. Try to find a private toilet where you can gag and cough up mucous as you spit the oil out. See tips below.

6. Rinse and gargle mouth and throat with a handful of water. This step is to rinse away some of the bacteria, chemicals, and parasites before sticking your toothbrush in your mouth.

7. Brush teeth and tongue well. Take your time brushing both your teeth and tongue. Remember, a ton of bacteria has been there, so you want to saturate the mouth and destroy them. Try to use a natural toothpaste to minimize chemical use. You can alternatively use a 50-50% combination of baking soda and sea salt to brush your teeth and tongue. Plain old baking soda will work very well too.

8. Drink one or two 8-oz glasses of water (always after brushing). This serves multiple purposes. Drinking a glass of water first thing in the morning can be both cleansing and liberating.

Sleep is a major way of detoxing the body. When you wake up, some bacteria will have risen to the surface overnight—chunks in the corners of eyes, dark/ bubbly first morning urine, foul breath. You just spent hours fasting and detoxing.

A great way of helping your body to come out of this detox phase is to drink a glass of water. It also rehydrates the body after hours of no water.

However, because we are doing our morning oil pulling routine, you should opt to drink your water *afterwards.* Another reason why we need to drink water after is to suspend any further oil pulling activity that your body feels the urge to do. Remember, your body just spent the last 15-20 minutes pulling stuff up. Downing water will give your body the subtle suggestion that it is time to stop. Further, you should always hydrate the body after a serious detoxification session. Drinking the water after brushing will help you feel good after your session.

9. Enjoy the benefits of oil pulling! And remember—keep on pulling. Once you get the hang of it, it will become second-nature to you and you will never want to go without!

When Is the Best Time to Oil Pull?

The morning is generally the best time to pull. **It is good to oil pull at least four hours after eating and at least one hour after drinking any beverages.** You may find greater success by building a morning routine, rather than trying to juggle oil pulling in between meals and drinks during the day and evening. Being too ambitious or creative with your oil pulling could lead to a sense of feeling overwhelmed, or feeling like you need to "squeeze it in," along with all the other stuff you have to do.

This may lead to stress, as you consider the whole spectrum of health, diet, fitness, and your other healthy commitments. Plus, it's plain confusing having to calculate all day.

So rather than thinking of when, and after what meal, or which glass of water, simply resolve to oil pull first thing in the morning. The perfect time is when you wake up, and before anything can mess up your day. Just roll out of bed and do it. Then there will be no question of what you've eaten, or whether you should take that sip of water. Banning yourself from water for an hour during the day could make you thirsty and anxious anyway.

A morning routine will be the best way to build your daily oil pulling habit. Furthermore, you will become absolutely addicted to the beautiful feeling of starting your day with minimal mucous in your nose, throat, and chest. Taking several long, deep, slow breaths after you pull will help you feel energized, as breathing is detoxifying as well.

Get It Out!

If you live with others and you have more than one toilet at home, use the toilet which is far from others so that you can be as loud as you need to be without being embarrassed. The best part about oil pulling is the end, so really cough it up.

Think of a dog, and how it automatically hacks when something really needs to come out. They don't mess around when they need something out immediately. If you are just innocently spitting into the toilet or trash bin in your best lady-like attempt, you will only get half the result! Follow these suggestions at the end of your oil pulling session:

- ❖ **Cough** it up.
- ❖ Do a **spastic, dog-like hack** with short, repeated coughs.
- ❖ **Gag.** Contract the back of your throat to squeeze out phlegm.
- ❖ **Snort** (not cocaine). Intake air noisily through the nostrils whilst gathering mucous.
- ❖ **Hock a Loogie**—Cough up a large globule of spit and slime.

Here are some useful do's and don'ts of oil pulling to help you achieve success with your oil pulling journey and your health.

The Do's of Oil Pulling Success

1. Do use top quality oils. The oils you select should accommodate your personal preference and cost, but you should always use cold-pressed, and organic whenever possible. The most popular oils to pull with are:

- ➢ Organic Cold-Pressed Sesame Oil (Not Toasted)
- ➢ Organic Extra Virgin Coconut Oil (Unrefined)
- ➢ Organic Extra Virgin Olive Oil

> Organic Cold-Pressed Sunflower Oil (Unrefined)

2. Do brush teeth after oil pulling. It is vital that you wash away the bacteria that has been pulled into the mouth. Choose the toothpaste you like best. Oil Pulling works to cleanse the body of chemicals, so you may want to go with a natural toothpaste or opt for plain baking soda. Use straight baking soda if you have thrush, or a 50-50 mixture of baking soda and sea salt.

3. Do drink water after brushing teeth. Water will help regulate your system and let your body know that the pulling stage is over. It will also hydrate and replenish the body after the detoxification period.

The Don'ts of Oil Pulling Success

1. Don't oil pull within 4 hours of eating and 1 hour of drinking any beverage. The idea is to bring up toxins from the throat, esophagus and organs. There are two possible explanations for this rule, and I don't plan on testing them out. The first is that if you consume food and water at the wrong time, you may upchuck or become nauseated. The second is that you may lose out on nutrients of that healthy food you just consumed, negating the beneficial effect of the meal. Either way, if you pull in the mornings, you won't have much problem adhering to this rule.

2. Don't drink water before you brush your teeth. If you drink water before cleaning your mouth, you will simply be re-consuming the exact parasites and chemicals you didn't want to have in the first place.

3. Don't swallow the oil. The oil contains bacteria that you do not want in your stomach. If you accidentally swallow a tiny bit, don't fret, and keep swishing. Then add on 2-3 minutes to your total time to compensate and to allow for recovery of the small swallowed amount.

4. Don't stop oil pulling. Being healthy is a never-ending journey that you will live by. Remember, there is no "Get Healthy Quick" scheme. Just do the best you can and don't stress. If you pull every day, you will begin to see changes after 1-2 months. It's okay to miss a single day. However, if you stop for an extended period, your benefits end. So, keep on! And enjoy the freshness and vitality of oil pulling.

Best Oils to Pull With

Perhaps one of the most frequently asked questions is, "Which oil should I use to oil pull?"

Here you'll find information on some of the advantages, as well as a couple disadvantages of pulling with coconut oil compared to sesame oil. Then you can decide whether you want to use coconut oil or another oil for your daily oil pulling routine. Most people who are anxious to get started will head to their kitchen to grab the extra-virgin olive oil to start with, and then move on to another oil later. Some say the olive oil can be a little pungent or dry, but you should decide for yourself.

When oil pulling first began, it started with the use of sesame oil, in India. An old Ayurvedic practice, sesame oil was touted as excellent for wiping out both bacteria and viruses. Oil pulling is big in India. When you see a huge sesame oil advertisement on the side of a bus, you know they're not messing around.

Dr. Bruce Fife's Contribution to Oil Pulling

When Dr. Bruce Fife released his informative books, "The Coconut Oil Miracle," and "Oil Pulling Therapy: Detoxifying and Healing the Body Through Oral Cleansing," the modern idea of oil pulling was born. He showed how coconut oil could be used to fight viral diseases and help keep bacteria out of the mouth and body.

Dr. Fife asserts that "all disease starts in the mouth," because the mouth is a passageway for virus, bacteria, and fungi into our bodies. He explained that the human mouth contains over 10 billion bacteria, and that bodily health depended greatly on oral cleanliness. He also revitalized the ideas of the Greek physician, Hippocrates, who believed that diseases could be reversed by taking care of the mouth. Hippocrates even pulled a decaying tooth once to cure a person of arthritis. It seems that the state of your mouth affects all parts of your body, since bacteria can enter the bloodstream through seriously infected gums and float to the heart, lungs, joints, or the brain.

On a happier note, the doctor said that teeth were whitened and the overall condition of the gums and mouth became healthier with the simple act of oil pulling. He recommended coconut oil specifically because it was cheaper and healthier than sesame, and tastes better.

Comparing Coconut Oil to Sesame Oil

Other research has concluded that the traditional sesame oil may be more effective at pulling toxins. But for certain, know that both oils are effective and that you should also factor how much you *like* each oil. Each has a distinct taste. Some people find the nuttier sesame oil more convenient because you can pour the oil. Others find the taste of coconut oil more palatable. Both oils contain an abundance of nutrients and antioxidants which fight cancer. They are both anti-viral and anti-bacterial.

Is it Sustainable?

The most important thing to think about when choosing oil is, "How likely am I to stick to this routine using this type of oil?"

In other words, consider which oil is sustainable for you and your own lifestyle and taste. Which oil will you be likely to keep oil pulling with? You will achieve the greatest health effect from oil pulling not by the type of oil you use, but rather, the *longevity* of your oil pulling. Most people that achieve results from oil pulling, ultimately pull for life.

How to Oil Pull with Coconut Oil

As you may already know, coconut oil carries a solid temperature when the room is chilly, but may melt quite some in the summer, depending on where you live. You do not need to microwave the coconut oil to get it to a liquid state. Instead, simply cut off a small chunk with a metal spoon, and place it in your mouth. Coconut oil will generally melt in your mouth after 30 seconds, and then you can proceed with swishing like normal.

Coconut Oil is Great for Other Uses Too

Another factor to consider is the one-jar-convenience of coconut oil. As you may know, coconut oil has many other uses beyond oil pulling. You can put coconut oil on your skin to create softness, put it in your hair to soften your tresses, and massage it into your scalp to help hair grow.

And of course, you can and should use extra-virgin unrefined coconut oil for cooking, as long as your food is cooking below 350° Fahrenheit or 177° Celsius. If you are boiling or simmering, temperature will reach only 212° Fahrenheit or 100° Celsius. This means you can use extra-virgin unrefined coconut oil in soups or stews.

However, if you use refined coconut oil, which Dr. Fife says is fine for oil pulling, you can cook food up to 450°. You will reach this temperature when frying food.

Frying food causes unwanted oxidation of food, as oil can reach high-heat temperatures of 350°-450°, so you should fry food sparingly. If you must fry, choose either refined coconut oil or avocado oil.

Sautéing is not the same as frying. Pan temperature is low enough for extra virgin unrefined coconut oil.

A Personal Word on Brands of Coconut Oil

I've experimented with my fair share of coconut oils. They do not all taste the same. I even remember tasting and immediately returning one to the supplier because I was sure it was rancid. I was embarrassed when they got back to me saying that they lab-tested it to check for mold and bacteria, and there was absolutely nothing wrong with it. It just didn't taste good to me.

My favorite coconut oil is Nutiva. I like the mildness of this coconut oil and it works well with my budget since I can buy it in bulk. The container is the perfect size for my kitchen because it's small enough to sit conveniently on my window sill, yet large enough to get a good deal on price. I like to keep it on my window sill because it keeps it a little warmer than our cold pantry. I use it for cooking and natural hair concoctions and it's fantastic. I also love that Nutiva is a sustainable organic company that cares about humanity and the planet.

Chapter Five

What About Side Effects?

Oil pulling does not really have any side effects, but you will probably experience the "Herxheimer Reaction" and "die-off" symptoms. The main premise behind this bodily reaction is that you may experience discomfort while bacteria is dying off and leaving your body. Note that these are not side effects, but rather, are a natural reaction to healthy change happening within the body. It's kind of like getting worse before getting better.

Herxheimer Reaction includes, but is not limited to the following:

- Feeling of a cold or flu
- Cysts or blisters
- Headache
- Nausea
- Generally achy or tired

The term "Herxheimer" comes from Dr. Karl Herxheimer, who was treating patients with syphilitic lesions. This German doctor noticed that patients who got the worst lesions, and who experienced fever, nausea and flu symptoms, recovered faster. Sure, their symptoms were hellish for 2-3 days, but then they healed.

This is exactly the type of approach you need to take with your oil pulling. Know that you may get "sick" in the beginning while your body is ridding itself of predators.

The bacteria and parasites will be happiest in their comfort zone, where they are tearing apart your body and feeding off of your supplies (your nutrients). When you break them away from their feeding frenzy, it disturbs them. Their dying within you can bring feelings of sickness and emotion. They release their toxins into your bloodstream, causing your body to prepare for sickness by creating an inflammatory response. A Herx reaction can be just as dramatic for a course of antibiotics as it can for a natural treatment.

Eliminate

Your elimination systems–your skin, kidneys, lungs, liver, and intestines will play a key role in how quickly you recover from your Herxheimer's reaction. If your elimination systems are working properly, you can expect to recover from a bout of Herxheimer's reaction within 1-10 days.

If your elimination system is not working well, try speeding it along with an enema or colon cleanse. Often times, our bodies and chosen remedies are busy working hard for us, but the last task at hand–the movement from your body to the toilet slows the process. Detoxing will quicken your recovery, while taking an anti-inflammatory like an ibuprofen pill will simply prolong recovery by masking pain.

Be sure to drink lots of water to rinse away bacteria, and also to get plenty of sleep to improve your bodily function.

How to Shorten Herxheimer Recovery Time

1. Drink plenty of fresh, clean water
2. Get extra deep, healing sleep to recuperate the body
3. Take Epsom Salt baths to release toxins

4. Do an enema
5. Get a deep tissue massage to release toxins
6. Drink detoxifying tea throughout the day

With oil pulling, newcomers specifically complain of nausea, cold/ flu, and cysts or blisters on the gums or elsewhere. This is a surefire sign that your oil pulling efforts are working. Cysts, blisters, and sores on the gums mean that the bacteria is rising to the surface. In this case, the body is using skin tissue as an elimination method. Your body is sending them to the nearest exit, instead of transporting it all the way through your digestive system.

Emotional Reactions

Perhaps some of the most interesting reactions are that of emotion. Many people believe that oil pulling relates only to oral health. However, after your mouth is healed, the healing will venture into other areas of your body that may need detoxification or healing. Different emotions may speak to you, depending on which organ is being cleansed. The chart below represents surfacing feelings during times of detoxification.

Emotion & Organ
Anger: Liver
Hatred: Liver
Melancholy: Liver
Bitterness: Pancreas
Envy: Abdomen
Fear: Kidneys
Grief: Thymus Gland
Guilt: Reproductive Organs

Sadness: Heart
Sorrow: Heart

The emotional reactions of detoxification can also be shortened by drinking water and getting plenty of rest. In addition to these, also try yoga poses which balance emotions.

Check out the Jumpstart Cleanse at the back of the book when you're ready to get started!

Sources

Anand T., Pothiraj C., Gopinath R.N, and B. Kayalvizhi. "Effect of Oil Pulling on Dental Caries Causing Bacteria." *Oil Pulling Secrets.* African Journal of Microbiology Research Vol.(2) pp.063-066, March, 2008.

Asokan S, Emmadi P, and Raghuraman Chamundeswari. "Effect of Oil Pulling on Plaque-Induced Gingivitis: A Randomized, Controlled, Triple-Blind Study." *Indian Journal of Dental Research.* 1 Oct 2008.

Asokan S, Rathan J, Muthu MS, Rathna PV, Emmadi P; Raghuraman; Chamundeswari. "Effect of Oil Pulling on Streptococcus Mutans Count in Plaque and Saliva using Dentocult SM Strip Mutans Test: a randomized, controlled, triple-blind study." *J. Indian Soc. Pedod Prev. Dent.* 2008 Mar;26(1):12-7.

"Coconut Oil Pulling—What the Wise Ones Do India." *Dr. Sarah Larsen.* n.d. Web 01 Dec 2013.

"Dherbs Detox Troubleshoot." *Dherbs.* , n.d. Web 14 Dec 2013.

Fife, Bruce. Oil Pulling Therapy: Detoxifying and Healing the Body Through Oral Cleansing. Colorado Springs, CO: Picadilly Books, 2008.

"Herxheimer Reaction." *Chronic Illness Recovery Counsel Liason Education.* Chronic Illness Recovery. 8 Sept 2014, Web.

Moncel, Bethany. "Smoking Point of Fats & Oils." *About.* IAC, n.d. Web. 14 Dec 2013.

"Oil Pulling has Cured...insert your story. THX!" *Cure Zone Oil Pulling Forum.* Web 1 Nov 2013.

Thaweboon S., Nakaparksin J., and Boonyanit Thaweboon. "The Effect of Oil Pulling on Oral Microorganisms in Biofilm Models." *Asian Journal of Public Health.* August 2011. 2(2): 62-66.

"The Herxheimer's Reaction---Feeling Worse Before Feeling Better." *Bioveda Welness.* BioLight Technologies, 10 Feb 2010, Web.

"User Experiences." *Oil Pulling. org.* Web 01 Nov 2013

Jumpstart Cleanse--BONUS

The purpose of this cleanse is not to starve you to death, but rather, to help you feel good by eliminating some of the dumb foods that wreak havoc on your body. Starving yourself would only put your body in to starvation mode, and then it would start to hoard fat. Instead, we want to limit NO foods, and load up on the YES list below.

By the end of this cleanse, you should feel lighter and more energetic. It is important to note that every body is different. Everybody is on a different stage in their health journey, and every individual body reacts differently. Feel free to modify this cleanse as much as you need to, but do not modify it to the point where you are cheating. Before you order that latte, think about your future self. Picture yourself getting up in the morning and looking in the mirror. The only person you have to answer to when following a self-guided program is the person in the mirror. What will you tell yourself in the morning? Will you like yourself tomorrow, or will you bad-mouth yourself for cheating?

The cleanse below has fairly simple guidelines and is not complicated to prepare for and follow. You may interchange foods on the YES list, but be sure to eat protein and veggies at every meal.

Oil pull every morning when you wake up. For this cleanse, we will oil pull using 2 drops of oil of oregano placed into ¾ tablespoon of coconut or sesame oil. If you are using a very hard coconut oil (due to the temperature of the room), you will need to heat the coconut oil VERY MINIMALLY in the microwave. Do not fully melt the coconut oil. Then mix 2 drops of oil of oregano into the coconut oil.

If you are using sesame oil, you only need to drop 2 drops of oil of oregano into your spoon of already-poured sesame oil. Use sesame oil if you want to avoid using the microwave.

Do not use oil of oregano without enveloping it into either coconut or sesame.

All foods should be bought organic and local whenever possible. If you shudder when you look at organic prices, try to at least opt for antibiotic-free meat and eggs, organic apples, organic spinach, and organic kale.

Drink 8-10 glasses of fresh filtered water per day.

YES
Lots of veggies
Fruits
All kinds of tea
1 whole egg + 2 egg whites per serving
4-6 oz. salmon per serving
4-6 oz. tuna per serving
20 unroasted, unsalted nuts, like almonds or walnuts
Raw seeds (pumpkin seeds fight parasites)
Stevia, unlimited
1 cup legumes per meal (NO soy)
Raw honey (But don't go overboard)
Extra virgin coconut oil, unlimited (but don't go cray-cray)
Extra virgin olive oil, unlimited (don't go cray-cray)
Avocado oil, unlimited (don't go cray-cray)

NO
Fatty meats
Soy (occasional soy sauce is fine)
Sugar & all its forms (no evaporated cane juice or other "healthy" sugars)
All Alcohol (Including wine and vodka)

Chips
Wheat (Imported European rye bread is fine, if you can get it)
White rice
Soda
Milk
Cheese
Peanuts
Processed food
Canola oil and Margarine
Coffee

All Days:
Awake, oil pull immediately
Drink 2 glasses of filtered water
Prepare green tea with the juice of one lemon plus raw honey or stevia

Breakfast:
Green Smoothie:
1 cup of UNSWEETENED almond milk
¼ cup raw seeds, like sunflower or pumpkin
1 cups greens, like spinach, kale, or dandelion greens
1 banana
½ cup fruit of your choice
Egg white or hemp protein powder (optional)
Blend all in blender

Snack:
Organic apple
20 raw almonds or walnuts

Lunch:

Lean protein from YES list
Large green salad
1-2 tbs. olive oil and lemon or lime salad dressing
¼ cup cooked brown rice OR
1 slice imported European rye bread

Snack:
Cut veggies
¼ cup guacamole

Dinner:
Lean protein from YES list
Large green salad with olive oil-lemon salad dressing OR
2 cups vegetable soup

This cleanse can be used all the time. Do it as much as you like or make it a permanent change. If this is already a typical eating day for you or you eat like this on most days, way to go! You may want to advance it further with some detoxifying herbs.

Last Thoughts

People are constantly searching for the miracle cure, or the magic pill that will solve their health issues for once and for all. Health does not work that way. Good health is about a long-term lifestyle, not a single simple action that can produce dramatic results within a few days.

Think of it like exercise. You must do it daily or at least a few times a week for the rest of your life. Walking or riding a bike for one week may have improved your health for that week, but you probably won't see results until you are far into your workouts. If you were to stop your daily exercise routine, the benefits would stop as well.

And just like exercise, you won't see drastic results in two weeks from oil pulling. Don't expect a miracle cure for psoriasis in two weeks, and don't expect to lose 10 pounds either. Oil pulling is not a sudden cure. It is part of a healthy way of life.

Also, like exercise, if you go pig out at the happy hour afterward, you can throw half your hard work and results out the window. If you haven't already done so, develop a whole lifestyle, equipped with exercise, clean eating, and a few other add-ons, like supplements, oil pulling, enemas, cleansing, and meditation.

What you will see is a gradual improvement in your health after 2-3 months, and a slow transition to health and healing. Everybody is different, and we all experience sickness and recovery differently. But making oil pulling part of your morning routine will contribute to your overall health. I promise that once you build an oil pulling habit, you will never want to go back to your old routine.

I'm so happy you picked up this book and that I could share one of my best health secrets with you. I hope you will use it to get started with a successful oil pulling journey. From my heart to yours—cheers to good health!

One Last Thing Before You Go

Thank you so much for purchasing this book and reading it. I hope you have enjoyed reading it as much as I have enjoyed writing it. I would be honored and grateful if you posted a review of this book and/or shared your thoughts of this book with your friends. It will help other readers find the book. They might want to be oil pullers too.

About the Author

Sonja Larsen is a health writer from Los Angeles who has travelled all over the world. She loves devouring healthy things, and has a fondness for oils and Mediterranean cuisine.

She is absolutely delighted that the digital age makes it possible for everyone to connect and share. But she does like to power down at the house every once in a while to sip some hot tea and chillax with an old-fashioned pen and paper.

Sonja loves people. Please contact her at sonjalarsen@live.com with questions or just to say hi.

Special Excerpt:

Oil Belly, Flat Belly
-Excerpt from Chapter 1, Abs are Made in the Kitchen-

The Hoarding of Fat

We are modern beings living in the same bodies as those who lived before us. Only now, we consume processed food-like substances, and we spin wheels to consume them faster.

When your body senses a shortage of food, it begins hoarding fat. This is the way we function. Humans survived and thrived this way before they could make a pit stop at the neighborhood market. We used to have to hunt or gather our meals. Now we just pass by the fast food drive-thru lane on the way home.

It was feast or famine for our ancestors, and their bodies adapted to ways of coping through times of famine. Perhaps a drought occurred, or a hunter returned with no meat. Maybe the ground was still frozen from winter, and food was hard to come by.

Your body responds to starvation by hoarding fat. It's your body's way of shutting down energy-burning until it is sure to receive the next meal. Your body is designed to miraculously survive for days from conserving energy in this manner. It conserves energy using two tactics:

The body stores energy as fat until food arrives, just in case more shortages occur. It remembers how bad it was last time it had to go without fuel.

The body decreases how much energy it spends, so that it will have enough energy to seek more food. It's like a signal that says, "Hey…slow that metabolism down for a while, until things get back to normal!"

These mechanisms will work beautifully if a natural disaster occurs or if we somehow sink into a national food shortage. But it wreaks havoc when we are trying to squeeze into a pair of skinny jeans.

Metabolism has two basic states: the catabolic state and the anabolic state. Catabolism is when your body is breaking down muscle. Anabolism is when your body is building muscle. Going for many hours without food can put your body in to a catabolic state, depending how much protein you ate in the last meal.

Perhaps the most likely catabolic state comes after skipping breakfast. You go 8 hours without eating while in bed, but then you don't eat breakfast--even though the point of breakfast is literally to break the fast.

In other words, you eat dinner at 7 pm. You go to bed and get up. You skip breakfast and just have lunch the following day at 12 noon. That's a whopping 17 hours without eating! Even a midmorning snack at 10 am would put you at 15 hours without eating. It's a double-whammy. Not only does your body begin feeding off your muscle for energy (cannibalizing itself), but it also begins hoarding fat.

In a 2004-2006 Australian research study[1], 2184 participants journaled their diets daily, with specific notation on whether they had eaten breakfast or not. Those who skipped breakfast were found to have larger waist circumferences (bigger bellies), and higher fasting insulin.

Low-calorie, low-fat dieting only aggravates the problem. When you try to use a low-calorie diet, you may just end up burning through muscle and storing fat. Dieting will not only trigger the fat-hoarding, but will slow your metabolic rate as well.

You may have heard fitness trainers use the word, "metabolic rate." The metabolic rate is the number of calories you would burn if you were at rest. It is how much energy you expend when you are not working out. If you think about it, you want to burn calories when you get out of the gym, not only when you're there. The treadmill is just a machine that counts calories while you are there, but the real magic happens when you are not running on it.

Another contributor to the hoarding of fat is the lack of fat intake. When you go on a fat-free or low-fat diet, your body says, "There will be no more fat coming. Hold on to that fat!"

When we eat good fats, we create movement which stimulates abdominal fat. Your old fat is stagnantly resting and needs to be urged to move. Stimulation is good. Stagnation is bad.

Some of the best oils will eliminate stagnation within your body, and the worst oils will "stick," to your body, causing horrific inflammation and cardiovascular disease.

Omega-3 fats are crucial to maintaining health and weight. We'll discuss omega-3 and omega-6 fatty acids in much more detail in Chapter 4. For now, know that one of the major problems with eating processed food is that the worst oils are commonly used—processed omega-6 oils. Most Western diets splurge on omega-6 foods like there's no tomorrow.

We need to eat as much omega-3 fats as possible to balance out our bad tendency to eat omega-6 fats. The omega-6 heavy-hitters are sunflower oil, canola oil, soybean oil, safflower oil, and anything you see labeled "vegetable oil" or "shortening." Stop putting these factory oils in to your cart. You'll find out why you need to avoid these oils in Chapter 5.

In a 2013 obesity study [43], scientists gave 6 grams of fish oil to one group and 6 grams of sunflower oil to the other group. Both groups walked 3 times per week for 45 minutes as a form of exercise. At the end of 4 weeks they found that their levels of omega-3 fatty acids, EPA and DHA were higher. Then they measured again after 8 weeks. They found a significant reduction in weight of the omega-3 fish oil group.

If you eat out often, you are most likely eating heavily processed food. You won't be able to control the type of oil you take in, nor the amount of oil. Find foods which you can prepare quickly at home. You don't always need to make cooking fancy. Trying to follow recipes from famous television chefs can lead to a sense of feeling overwhelmed in the kitchen. Often, gourmet chefs aim to impress others with their exotic culinary skills, rather than showing us how to make basic, everyday food. Daily cooking does not need to be a big project.

Prepare simple foods, and make them in abundance so that you'll have food for a couple days. Go raw sometimes—it's quicker. Get a slow cooker with a delay timer. Then you will be able to eat at home more often. If you are stretched for time one day, shop at the deli/hot foods section of the health food market. Many health food markets carry to-go-meals with the exact ingredients listed. Some even have seating areas. However, eating prepared foods from health food stores can be pricey, so you may want to use this option only when you need to order food out.

Read the following list. Limit foods from the "Bad Fats" list, and eat foods from the "Good Fats" list daily...

-Oil Belly, Flat Belly

Made in the USA
Las Vegas, NV
22 June 2022